YOUR
Fat Loss Forever
Guide

The Secret to Lasting Weight Loss, More Energy, Less Pain, & Optimized Hormonal Health

Bradley Goins- Certified Personal Trainer
Jessica Goins- RN, Health Coach

First Printing: 2018

ISBN-13: 978-1-7326312-0-5

www.goinsstrong.com

Table of Contents

"If we could give every individual the right amount of nourishment and exercise, not too little, and not too much, we would have found the safest way to health."

– Hippocrates

"The secret of change is to focus all of your energy, not on fighting the old, but on building the new."

– Socrates

"The doctor of the future will give no medication, but will interest his patients in the care of the human frame, diet and in the cause and prevention of disease."

– Thomas A. Edison

"If you look closely, most overnight successes took a long time."

– Steve Jobs

"Knowing is not enough; we must apply.
Willing is not enough; we must do."

– Johann Wolfgang von Goethe

Introduction

Welcome to "Your Fat Loss Forever Guide", the last "diet" book or guide you will ever need; because it is based in science and personally tested through application!

My name is Bradley Goins. I am co-owner of Goins Strong Fitness in Dallas, NC with my beautiful wife Jessica. The health and fitness arena has become a calling for both of us.

Jessica has a background as a Registered Nurse and as a certified Health Coach. I am a certified Personal Trainer and have dedicated my life to health, fitness, and helping others. (I am also a degreed Electrical Engineer, but that's a different story).

Between us, we have over 30 years of fitness experience and application, including group instruction and leading our own fitness business. We have two amazing young boys, ages 6 and 1 (as I write this).

This document is our collective effort to bring you a comprehensive guide that enhances your life.

I became obsessed with fitness and health at the age of 14 (roughly 18 years ago). Prior to that I had struggled with childhood obesity.

At my worst, I recall weighing 140 pounds when I was a little over 4 feet tall around 10 years of age.

My Body Mass Index (BMI) was well over 30 (clinically obese). During this time, I also struggled with chronic asthma!

Had things not changed for me, my life would have been much different.

At a young age, I discovered weight training, and like a sponge, I soaked up every piece of knowledge I could find on diet and exercise.

I began to apply it in my own life. I didn't have a "mentor", or a "trainer". My doctor couldn't provide the advice I needed. I was on my own!

I've spent years sorting through blogs, articles, studies, and experimenting with different "diets" and training methods.

I took action by experimenting on myself, in hopes that I could gain enough experience to help as many others as possible.

No one, should have to suffer from obesity and other related illnesses.

No one, should feel like a prisoner in their own bodies.

Everyone should have the knowledge to build the body of a Greek statue! If that is their desire.

EVERYONE is worthy of the FREEDOM that comes from good health!

Along this journey, I have gained perspectives on what works and what doesn't.

Because of this journey, I am now positioned to help you and anyone who lays hands on this document.

In this guide, lies our collective perspective on "Diet", and how you should approach it.

We have worked to make the information as simple and readable as possible.

This is not a doctoral level thesis on nutrition or the psychology of lifestyle change.

It is written such that ANY man, woman, or child could take the information and USE IT!

After all, what is the point of good information if people can't understand and apply it?

This isn't your typical "how to count calories" or "keep track of your macros" guide.

This guide is solely based on the hormonal effects of food in the body. We'll help you take back control of your body!

You will be armed with powerful information that will help you understand WHY certain foods are better choices than others.

I have condensed 15+ years of study and application into as few pages as possible. This isn't just a guide, I consider it my life's work.

Had I never applied the information contained here, I would have never met my wife, and therefore would not have my wonderful children…

I would have never built the life destined for me.

Without the confidence gained from better health, I wouldn't have believed in myself enough to attend college in the field of Electrical Engineering. I wouldn't have had the mental fortitude required to persevere through school when it truly got difficult.

By extension, I would not have been positioned to obtain a good job in a technical field and provide for my family.

And without financial stability gained from my technical job, I would not have been able to fund the opening of our gym; and therefore, would not be in a position to help YOU!

I owe my current existence to my past self. I thank that young teenager every day.

What if he had ignored that voice calling from deep inside? What if he had never made a change?

How would my current life be different, now?

SO... before we dive into this life changing information, let me summarize with this...

Your FUTURE self depends on your PRESENT self!

Don't let YOU down!

If at any point you struggle to apply this information in your own life, **we are here for you!**

Come by and see us at **Goins Strong Fitness** in Dallas, NC. If you are not local, and remote coaching is something you feel you need, we will work to make sure you are successful…

Reach out to us by email:

jessica@goinsstrong.com **OR** bradley@goinsstrong.com

How Food Affects the Body:

Why Blood Sugar and Insulin Control Are the Keys Behind Every Popular "Diet"
(Part 1)

I'm going to let you in on a little secret… "Diets work"!

Though, it's not because any particular diet is the "holy grail". The reason most diets work (at least while you are on them) is because nearly every popular diet recommends reducing and eliminating as much highly processed food as possible (i.e. sugar, soda, bread, etc.).

If you eat a highly processed "American" diet, and switch to a natural whole-food based diet…You will typically see results very quickly.

Usually you will feel much better as well, since you have started feeding yourself real food instead of processed flour and sugar!

You have likely heard of "Low-Carb", "No-Carb", "Paleo", "Atkins", "Ketogenic", "Zone", "Carnivore", "Vegan", "Vegetarian".

Each of these diets have their own nuances that make them slightly different and everyone screams about how their diet is the best.

There is no doubt that certain diets have reasons why they may be better than others. There are certain principles that make these diets effective.

Here is the main one:

They control blood sugar and insulin! [1] [2]

Forget all the extra marketing, and buzz words. Ignore the cult like behavior of ***some*** Vegans (If they promote high protein intake they're ok).

Blood sugar and insulin control are the main drivers of these "diets"!

As a specific example of why insulin control matters, consider this… Insulin therapy commonly results in weight gain in both Type 1 and Type 2 Diabetes. This weight gain can be excessive, adversely affecting cardiovascular risk profile. [2]

If insulin therapy has this effect on diabetics…

Why are non-diabetics any different?

Guess what...They are not!

Excessive insulin inhibits the body's natural ability to regulate weight.

Therefore, the secret behind 'fat loss', 'good health', 'clearer thinking', 'fighting disease'…

Is as simple as choosing only foods that cause no or slow increases in blood sugar…

This keeps the body from releasing excessive amounts of insulin (The Storage Hormone).

Quick Lesson [3][4]

Insulin is a major hormone released by the pancreas that regulates how your body utilizes carbs, fat, and protein. It helps your muscles, liver, and fat cells process and utilize glucose (aka blood sugar).

Whenever we eat, our blood sugar goes up (mostly driven by carbohydrate consumption), our body responds by releasing an amount of insulin dependent on the type and amount of food we have consumed.

Insulin then uptakes the blood glucose and uses what it can for immediate energy usage, and any excess is stored in the muscles, liver, and fat cells. This is all part of how our bodies work to maintain a normal balance.

Different foods cause different increases in blood sugar and insulin – some higher, some lower. (We will get back to this later.)

Carbohydrates, especially sugar and processed grains will make blood glucose go up the most. Thus, a major insulin response follows.

Protein does cause a very slight insulin response, but there is little or no increase in blood sugar. (This is why many have found high protein, lower carb diets to be very effective for fat loss and reducing or eliminating diabetes medication…)

The American Diet has exploded into a huge problem in regards to "blood sugar and insulin control". Sugar and processed carbohydrates have become a "normal" part of the daily diet.

And while I certainly empathize with anyone struggling with weight (I have been there myself), these processed foods are slowly destroying us.

The rate of disease we are experiencing now, has never been seen in the history of the world. Why?

Because the easy and abundant access to processed food keeps us in a state where we are continually spiking our blood sugar.

Cereal and juice at breakfast…chips, soda, and sweets throughout the day. The body is not meant for this, and excessive increased blood sugar eventually leads to:

- Insulin resistance [7]
- Obesity and cardiovascular/heart disease that comes with it [5]
- Inflammation of arteries and veins (vascular system) [5]
- Cognitive decline (contributing to Alzheimer's and Dementia) [6]
- Poor energy levels

Your body does not want, nor is it designed to have excess sugar in the blood.

Why do you think it works so hard to regulate it?

A high level of blood sugar over time, eventually leads to Insulin Resistance.

This means your body's cells STOP properly responding to elevated insulin levels. This forces the body to release more insulin to produce a normal effect.

That means, you store MORE FAT (Insulin is the Storage Hormone).

In this state, you have created an environment where your metabolism stays in a "fat storage" mode.

This is why so many people struggle to lose weight.

Staying in a prolonged state of insulin resistance with consistently high blood sugar will eventually lead to the development of Type 2 Diabetes.

Many people wait until the doctor tells them they have diabetes before ever trying to fix their lifestyle.

YOU can and MUST take control much sooner!

Long before anyone becomes diabetic, they are doing damage to their cardiovascular system due to the vascular inflammation that comes from a poor diet and body composition. [5]

Waiting to do something about this is like playing Russian Roulette…

Eventually the chamber is loaded when you pull the trigger.

Take control now and live the life you're meant to…free of sickness and disease.

Now, let's dive deeper into the causes of obesity and insulin resistance…

How Fructose (and excess carbohydrates) are the ROOT CAUSE of Obesity!

As discussed already, when we consume carbohydrates our pancreas releases insulin to shuttle blood glucose to various cells in the body.

Insulin acts as a "key" to these cells. Insulin (the key) unlocks a "doorway" to the cell allowing blood glucose to flow in to be used as energy.

If you consume more sugar than the body needs, insulin will help store it in the liver, muscle cells, and fat cells; to be used when your blood sugar drops between meals.

Here's the important part…

Liver and Muscle cells have a limit to how much glucose they can store. Fat cells do NOT!

This means that when your muscle cells and liver are full, the majority of excess glucose will be forced into your fat cells! Not good if you are working hard to lose fat, right?

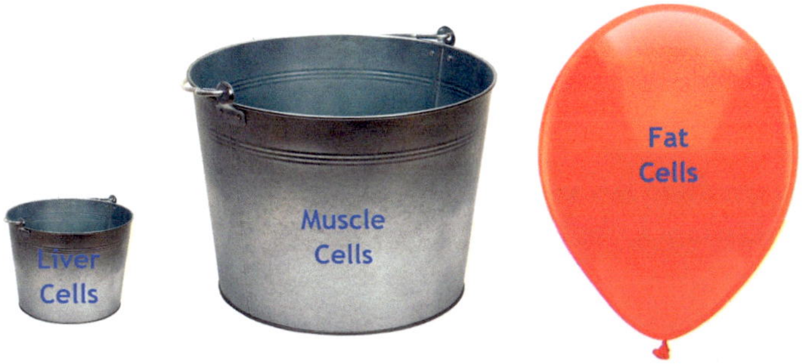

If you have a very high sugar/carbohydrate diet most days, you are keeping the liver and muscle buckets FULL; and likely stuffing many of the carbs you're eating into your fat cells (blowing up that balloon)!

This reduces your body's ability to burn existing body fat, as well!

Think of this constant consumption of sugar and simple carbohydrates like continuously filling up a car's gas tank (even though it is already full).

You are adding gasoline (sugar/carbs) for energy use many times per day, and your body never gets a chance to switch over to use your fat cells! (Keeping you in FAT STORAGE mode!)

Understanding the storage capacity of your individual body and the glycemic index (explained later) of your carbohydrate sources is important to managing your weight, FOREVER!

A ripped male bodybuilder will have a lot more muscle cells for storage (bigger bucket), than a smaller sedentary woman (smaller bucket). He therefore, can get away with eating a higher carbohydrate diet.

Additionally, this bodybuilder has trained his body to be extremely efficient at storing carbohydrates in the muscle cells.

He is weight training several times per week, and the higher carbohydrate diet he follows can work well for him (and also because he has virtually no insulin resistance).

Sedentary individuals, who are not weight training this intensely, DO NOT have the same ability to process a higher carbohydrate diet.

They are not active enough to burn or efficiently store excess carbs in the same way!

Similarly, individuals who are already overweight will have some level of insulin resistance, making it harder to properly process ingested sugars and carbs.

Now that you understand how and where the body stores unused carbohydrates (glucose), let's get to the key point of this section…

Excess Fructose and Sugar consumption, is the main cause of insulin resistance, which leads to obesity!

One study identified that "Consuming fructose-sweetened, not glucose sweetened beverages increases visceral adiposity and lipids [*Fat Gain*] and decreased insulin sensitivity [*Increased Insulin Resistance*] in over-weight/obese humans". [7]

I want to point out that everyone in this study GAINED fat, but only the 'fructose' group became more insulin resistant. WHY? Simple…

Fructose bypasses the muscle cells (the larger bucket) and is processed **only** by the liver. The liver has the smallest capacity (smaller bucket).

You can see how quickly the liver bucket will fill up when consuming high amounts of fructose. [8]

Guess what happens when that liver bucket is full? YUP! Your fat cells get a feeding frenzy!

On the other hand, glucose (and foods that breakdown to glucose) can be utilized by every cell in the body. This means all the buckets can be used for storage.

Excess fructose will easily be stored as fat in the liver and body. This is how one can develop fatty liver, insulin resistance, and ultimately obesity and diabetes.

> **NOTE:** Insulin resistance means your body's cells no longer respond to a 'normal' amount of insulin. Think of the cell doorway/key example from earlier.
>
> Normal insulin (the key) levels no longer fully opens the cell's door. (Imagine the door as 'partially' open.) The body has become "resistant" to normal insulin levels. (The key doesn't work.)

In response to this, the body must produce more insulin (extra keys) to allow the cell doorway to properly open all the way.

Over time, chronic insulin resistance will lead to obesity and Diabetes (Type II).

In the study cited above, insulin resistance increased after only '8 weeks'.

Imagine what happens over the course of a decade?

Is it any wonder the rates of obesity and diabetes have sky rocketed over the last several decades?

This information indicates that a major part of preventing and reversing insulin resistance, obesity, and diabetes is to **AVOID fructose and sugar as much as possible.**

Fructose is a common food additive, because it is actually low on the Glycemic Index. It is often described as "diabetic friendly" because of this, but as outlined earlier, fructose is NOT your friend.

Here are the most common items to avoid…

1. High **fructose** corn syrup (read labels, it's in everything)
2. Sugar (Table sugar is about 55% fructose/45% glucose)
3. Fruit juice (& excessive amounts of natural or dried fruits)

These are just a few considerations. 1 & 2 are pretty obvious, yet many people simply don't pay attention to the food labels.

Many so called "healthy" foods like Honey Nut Cheerios (and other cereals), yogurt, wheat bread, etc.…all contain added sugar and/or high fructose corn syrup.

Start reading the label to become aware of what is in your food!

Fruit is natural but does have high levels of natural fructose. The body doesn't care where the fructose comes from, even if it is a healthy fruit!

Fruit juice has had all the fiber removed, leading to faster digestion and larger insulin response.

It is also very easy to over consume fruit sugar in liquid form.

(No one needs to put a whole apple, pear, and banana in one smoothie…This is way too much fructose!)

We're not saying to never have fruit, but you must account for these facts.

If your goal is fat loss or if you are insulin resistant or diabetic; you will want to keep fruit consumption to a minimum.

Now, you are likely thinking…

> "What am I supposed to do?" …
>
> "I have eaten this way for many years, and struggle to lose weight"…
>
> "You're telling me I've been lied to my entire life about food?" …
>
> "And that even if I'm not diabetic, I most likely have some level of insulin resistance?"

YES! That is exactly what I am saying!

We have been lied too! The Food Pyramid was a harmful sham!

Doctors have told you to follow this same harmful information!

They will deny it, but…It's TRUE!

BUT, here is the GOOD NEWS…

ALL OF THIS IS PREVENTABLE & REVERSIBLE!!!

[Disclaimer: I want to clearly state that we are not doctors and that we are not "prescribing" a specific diet plan for any medical issue you may have. We do have many years of experience and application and are merely sharing our views on "diet" and the mindset you should have towards them.]

The cure for ALL this starts with **lifestyle change** (adjusting your habits).

Primarily, making optimal food choices and following a targeted exercise program (like the Goins Strong Fitness training classes)!

No magic pill can fix this...But YOU can!

A diet that controls "blood sugar" and "insulin" is the key to reversing insulin resistance, losing fat, and living longer!

This isn't a "diet" per say, **it's a LIFESTYLE**! It is based upon whole, nutrient-rich foods. A quality diet should consist of the following:

- Red meat, fish, poultry, eggs
- Vegetables (limited starchy)
- Dairy products (cottage cheese, Greek yogurt (unsweetened), most cheeses, etc.)
- Legumes
- Fruit
- Nuts
- Healthy fat sources (olive oil, coconut oil, natural butter, fish oil supplement)
- Some grains (limited 'low glycemic')

Simply stated, eat tons of protein (meat) and veggies, and enjoy some extra healthy fats. Fill up on these as much as possible.

Then enjoy ***some*** whole fruit if desired. Eat only small amounts of 'low glycemic' grains that supports physical activity (but not much beyond that).

[If fat loss is your primary objective, or you have an auto immune issue, grains should be avoided as much as possible]

A quick word about **Protein**…

So not only is protein great because of its very low impact on blood sugar and insulin, but it is the building blocks of our bones, muscles, tissues, hormone production and much more.

Some people have a fear that large amounts of protein will cause weight gain or bulky muscles. This is not true. Protein is essential for everyone, no matter age, gender, or activity level.

Unless you have a severe kidney issue already, do not worry about consuming higher amounts.

Higher intake is not linked to kidney issues in healthy individuals. Societies with high intake of meat (Japanese/Alaskan Inuits) have never suffered a rash of kidney problems.

What is important to note is the **amounts** of protein needed are different for each individual's **goals**. Though, there isn't truly an upper limit to what can be digested.

Also, Protein is not easily stored as body fat (which is why low-carb, Ketogenic type diets have been affective for many).

Short discussion on **Fat**…

Fats are essential for your body and proper hormone production, despite a decades long campaign against it. A 'low fat' diet is NOT good for you.

All fats are not created equal. You want to consume healthy fats from nuts and seeds (like hemp and chia), avocados, and egg yolks.

For cooking, use coconut oil, olive oil, or real butter.

Eat wild fish like 'wild' salmon (not farm raised), which is rich in Omega-3. Consider supplementing with a fish oil supplement, as most people do not or cannot get enough through diet alone.

Omega-3 is extremely important for brain health, fighting inflammation, and optimizing hormone levels. Also, high intake is linked to lower risk of heart disease.

Avoid the following fat sources, as they are highly inflammatory to the body:

- Soybean oil
- Vegetable oil
- Canola oil
- Margarines
- Corn oil
- Hydrogenated oils
- Safflower oil

(READ the food labels, as these are the most common oils used in the food industry because they are cheap.)

Glycemic Index Discussion

Now, let's talk about the Glycemic Index.

We've discussed the general idea of how the body processes carbohydrates via insulin release, let's get you up to speed on what the "Glycemic Index" is and how you can use it to your advantage.

The Glycemic Index (GI) is a measure of the effect carbohydrates have on blood glucose levels.

Understanding this will prevent harmful spikes in blood sugar, as sugars and carbohydrates are broken down and your pancreas releases insulin to use and/or store this blood glucose.

Limiting your intake of high GI foods is a first-step towards controlling cravings, increasing energy, and fat loss.

The Glycemic Index is based on the **quality** of carbohydrates and sugars you are eating, not the quantity. Carb-free foods such as meats and some vegetables have no (or very low) GI value.

Foods with a low GI (scores of 0-54) help you **feel less hungry**, **more energetic**, and will help you **burn more fat**.

Not to mention greatly reduce risk of diabetes and improve heart health (and overall health).

Note however, the AMOUNT you eat of these still matters.

Foods with a high GI score create a fast, sharp spike in insulin. This leads to more cravings shortly after you've eaten.

Ever eaten a high carb or sugar meal, only to find yourself starving a few hours later?

This is because you have crashed from the large blood sugar increase and insulin dump that occurred to bring your blood sugar back down (the crash).

In Part 3 of this guide, we list foods that are low on the Glycemic Index to assist you in your food choices.

In addition to the glycemic index rating we need be aware of the Glycemic 'Load' of the food we eat.

The glycemic load takes into account both the glycemic index of the food AND the **AMOUNT** of carbohydrate for a given serving.

What is the difference between Glycemic Index (GI) and Glycemic Load (GL)?

Your blood glucose rises and falls when you eat a meal containing carbs. How high it rises and how long it remains high depends on the quality of the carbohydrates (the GI) and the quantity (the serving size). Glycemic load or GL combines both the quality and quantity of carbohydrate in one 'number'. It's the best way to predict blood glucose values of different types and amounts of food.

Part 1 Summary for You:

Eat tons of meat (protein) and veggies to help you stay full and satisfied.

Choose carbohydrate sources that are **Low to Moderate** on the Glycemic Index.

Then also be aware of the **AMOUNT** of carbohydrates you are consuming (serving size).

Don't overwhelm yourself by overthinking the science behind it all.

OVER TIME, you will gain a better understanding as all this information sinks in.

Like a child learning to ride a bike, things can be difficult, because it is brand **new to you.** Soon you'll be riding that bike in the Tour De France!

Stay the course and continue to learn…

Think **long-term** and NEVER get discouraged! Re-read this information until it starts to make more sense!...

Your Attack Plan to Take Back Your Health

[How to Reverse Insulin Resistance]
(Part 2)

1. Make Protein the Base of Your Meals and Snacks

It is so important to take in adequate amounts of protein. Even if you are sedentary, you will greatly benefit from increasing your protein intake. [9]

When you are eating your meals and/or snacks, make sure to eat ALL of the protein to help you stay satisfied.

We personally do best when consuming 1 gram of protein per pound of body weight (150 lbs = 150+ grams), especially when weight training. This helps you to never feel hungry!

2. Avoid Sugar, Flour, and Refined/Processed Food

This will be the BIGGEST change you can make for your health. If you have a diet high in these products, removing them is the single greatest thing you can do for your LIFE!

You will feel so much better. I personally have had a significant reduction in joint pain, by completely eliminating these foods from my diet.

These are the foods and beverages that are "Killing America"!

Take back control of your health by removing these foods and replacing them with natural whole foods, we have conveniently listed out for you in Part 3.

Even if you are extremely active and appear healthy on the out-side, these foods still cause major issues for you internally.

Vascular inflammation isn't usually noticed until you end up in the hospital getting open heart surgery.

Take control now, by removing these foods from your diet…

Your future self will thank you!

3. Lift Weights to Build Muscle (Start with body-weight exercise if necessary)

This is known to increase insulin sensitivity (reduce insulin resistance) and increase metabolism.

It should be a tool in your belt to fight aging and disease. If your goal is fat loss, or just better health; you will be more successful if you start a dedicated weight training plan.

Many people think they should lose weight before they start weight training, or that cardio is the most important exercise for 'fat loss'…THIS IS FALSE!

Weight training will get you results faster. It revs up your metabolism and stimulates the body to produce more lean muscle mass.

All this helps you burn fat much faster!

Start with bodyweight squats and push-ups every day. Start wherever your current ability allows. DO NOT WAIT!

Reach out to us at Goins Strong Fitness and we will help get you started!

4. Eat Low Glycemic Carbs and Try to TIME Intake Near Training (When most active)

Follow the list of sources we have provided as much as possible.

Eat your carbs around training sessions or the most active times of the day. Minimize intake on the days you don't train (especially if your goal is fat loss).

This helps to ensure you keep the storage "buckets" of the muscle and liver cells from overflowing.

5. Get More SLEEP (7-9 hours)

Sleep affects ALL hormone production in the body, including insulin.

Make sure you get a 'minimum' of 6 hours a night, but preferably 7-9.

Getting good sleep is essential for recovery, reducing stress, and sense of well-being.

Skip sleep and you are playing a losing battle, so go to bed!

6. Perform Extra CARDIO in Combination with Your Weight Training

It's good for overall health and circulation. Get some Interval training / High Intensity Cardio often (2+ times/week).

This is built into our training classes at Goins Strong Fitness. We have witnessed the benefits of this training style in many individuals.

We have seen significant changes in individuals who weight train along with interval training only 2 times per week.

2 days per week is the perfect start. Results can come faster with 3-4, but 2 will create a dramatic change in your health!

In addition to the metabolic effects, this type of training is shown to increase insulin sensitivity, just like weight training.

This makes for a powerful combination in your fat-loss and long-term weight management goals.

7. Manage Stress in Your Life (Mental/Physical/Emotional)

Chronic stress can have a negative impact on your fat-loss goals. Excessive stress can lead to negative hormonal effects, such as elevated Cortisol levels in the body.

Too much Cortisol in the body, can inhibit your body from performing optimally; and directly impact any fat-loss goals.

Your 1st line treatments for "stress", are:

- Quality Whole Food Diet, as we outline in this guide (Natural food is medicine)
- Quality Sleep (Your body heals while you sleep)
- Regular Exercise (This helps the body become efficient in dealing with stressors)

The above have already been covered, but here's the next step:

Remove negativity from your life (Easier said, than done…I know!)

If something or someone causes you excessive emotional stress, it's time to cut it or them out of your life for a while!

I understand this isn't always possible, so it's important for you to understand that you can't control everything, BUT…

You CAN control how you "react" to it!

Avoid becoming emotional! Turn off the news, stop negative self-talk, avoid negative people…

Pay attention to how much better you feel when you do ALL of these things!

We cover this in more detail in the "Train your MINDSET for Lasting Success" bonus section.

8. Consider Berberine and Fasting as Additional Weapons

Fasting is something many people are scared of. We've been brainwashed that we MUST eat 6 times per day or our metabolism will slow down.

I can tell you from experience this advice is garbage…

I regularly practice Intermittent fasting as part of my normal life-style and have been happy with the benefits (clear thinking, staying leaner, reduced cravings).

In the BONUS #4 section, we've provided you a full discussion on Intermittent Fasting if you decide to give it a try!

Now, let's talk about Berberine!

This is a natural herbal supplement which originates from Chinese medicine. It has been found in studies to be as effective as the diabetes medication "Metformin".

That is pretty significant. It is rare that an herbal supplement is found to be this effective in an actual study.

I personally have added this to my supplementation plan due to its various benefits. (Research for yourself and discuss with your doctor any potential interactions with other medications you are taking.)

Berberine has anti-inflammatory and anti-fungal properties much like Turmeric (Curcumin) and has a significant impact in helping your body regulate blood sugar.

If you are overweight, remember you have some level of insulin resistance already, so Berberine could be a useful tool to assist in reducing insulin resistance and losing weight!

In the BONUS #3 section (Supplements Guide) we share additional information on Berberine.

Part 2 Parting Message:

You may have failed in the past, but **I PROMISE** you that if you follow a lifestyle of "blood sugar and insulin control" YOU WILL…

- Achieve a leaner body!
- Have more energy!
- Obtain improved hormonal health!
- Gain better quality of life!

How far you go is up to you. This is a **long-term** investment in yourself.

You do NOT need to be 'perfect'. You only need to start!

Try to make one change in the beginning.

Maybe give up sugary drinks like soda and juice (usually our biggest recommendation). We've seen people lose 30+ lbs by making that one single change.

Never get discouraged. This is not an 'all or nothing' plan.

If you have a bad meal, that's okay; this is about having a long-term mindset and making better choices.

You are not what you eat for one day, you are the average of what you eat over many days and years!

You CAN do it!

Foods to ENJOY!

(Part 3)

PROTEINS

Whole eggs	Liver
Beef	Bison
Chicken	Veal
Turkey	Duck
Lamb	Ostrich
Pork	Cottage cheese
Wild fish (not farm raised)	Yogurt (no sugar added)
Shell fish (shrimp, lobster, crab, etc.)	Whey protein powder

VEGETABLES

Leafy greens and lettuces	Mushrooms
Collards	Cauliflower
Spinach	Brussel sprouts
Broccoli	Artichoke
Kale	Alfalfa sprouts
Chard	Green beans
Cabbage	Celery
Onions	Radishes
Watercress	Garlic
Turnip	Scallions
Asparagus	Ginger
Parsley	Tomatoes (technically a fruit)
Okra	Bell peppers
Cucumbers	Egg plant
Zucchini	Snap peas

LOW GLYCEMIC STARCHES

(Consumed in small amounts)

Whole oats (not instant)	Sweet potato
Rice (brown, wild)	Peas
Beans (black, pinto)	Lentils
Quinoa	Sprouted grain bread (Ezekiel Bread)

FRUITS (Whole, not blended; Consumed in small amounts)

Berries (Blueberry, Strawberry, etc.)	Oranges
Grapefruit	Pears
Apples	Plums
Peaches	Grapes
Cantaloupe	Watermelon

SWEETNERS

(Limited - Used as a tool to reduce sugar intake)

Stevia (best option)	Splenda

FATS (Consumed in small amounts)

Olive oil	Natural butter
Coconut oil	Fish oil supplement
Avocado	Nuts / Chia & Hemp seeds

***This is not an all-inclusive list. It's simply a list of most common foods.**

Our Views on Low-Carb and Ketogenic Lifestyles

I wanted to add a section to specifically talk about this subject. We sometimes get asked our opinion on low-carb style diets, so we feel the need to clearly outline our views and why we hold them.

If you can't tell from the rest of this document…

WE LOVE LOW-CARB!

Why? Because Low-Carb and Ketogenic diets work! They work very well!

I personally follow a very low-carb diet when my primary goal is fat-loss. I have done this for many years, because fat-loss happens 2-3x times faster than when I try to get leaner on a higher carb diet.

I don't care what any doctor or nutritionist says. (Many are starting to recommend low carb diets for various issues.)

I have experienced the benefits myself and seen the results of others.

I never recommend anything I haven't done myself or have extensively researched to the point I can provide an informed position.

My joint pain is remarkably lower when I follow a low-carb, whole food diet.

My knee arthritis improves so much that going for a long run becomes possible.

If I stray too far from a controlled diet, inflammation flares back up making the thought of a run unbearable.

The medical community is slowly catching on, but if you are waiting for the medical field to recommend a low carb or ketogenic diet…You won't have it any time soon.

It's arguable that Protein and Fat are the only 'essential' macronutrients, and carbs are 'non-essential', since technically the body has the ability to produce needed glycogen via the liver.

(By the process of gluconeogenesis – The formation of glucose/glycogen from non-carbohydrate sources)

This is the premise behind low carb and Ketogenic diets.

I encourage you to search the internet for success stories of individuals who have changed their lives by switching to a low-carb or Ketogenic way of eating.

People who have struggled with weight their whole lives have found sudden success.

You'll find thousands of stories and accounts of individuals who have corrected many 'autoimmune' or inflammatory diseases by going to a low-carb, whole food diet.

As I mentioned, I personally found significant relief from the knee pain from my past injuries.

Many people with Type II Diabetes have come off or reduced their medications by following a low-carb protocol. The mechanism by which this happens is as we have described earlier in this guide…

Recall the "bucket" example we outlined. When you cut carbs to a low level, the glycogen "buckets" are able to drain.

The body must then dip more into the fat cells (balloon example).

The absence of carbs allows the body to utilize more stored energy from fat cells (deflating the balloon).

To be clear, the body is always using some stored fat for energy needs; however, a low-carb diet simply forces your body to 'oxidize' stored fat at a faster rate.

Additionally, if you are overweight, you already have some level of insulin resistance or pre-diabetes (it just hasn't become a major health issue yet).

A low-carb diet takes insulin out of the equation, by lowering its presence in the body.

As you recall, insulin resistance means your cells cannot properly respond to insulin.

By reducing insulin in your body and promoting a more efficient atmosphere for fat loss; the body can begin to heal itself.

Essentially, your body gets a break from insulin allowing it to slowly bring itself back into a normal balance.

To summarize, I recommend a low-carb diet to anyone who wants to optimize their ability to **burn fat**.

If you have struggled with 'lower calorie' diets before and failed, I highly recommend you look into a low-carb diet (this is not a 'low calorie' diet and you will not suffer severe hunger pains like you have in the past).

It may be the jumpstart you need to reverse years of built up insulin resistance.

This is a personal decision. If this is something you want to know more about, reach out to Jessica and me at Goins Strong Fitness.

Our mission is to end the cycle of Yo-Yo dieting…

We want you to WIN the WAR for your health!

REFERENCES

[1] Genetic Evidence That Carbohydrate-Stimulated Insulin Secretion Leads to Obesity

Published: January 2018

http://clinchem.aaccjnls.org/content/64/1/192

[2] Insulin-associated Weight Gain in Diabetes – Causes, Effects, and Coping Strategies

Published: 2007

www.Ncbi.nlm.nih.gov/m/pubmed/17924864

[3] ACE Essentials of Exercise Science for Fitness Professionals

ISBN 978-1-890720-58-2

Copyright 2010, 2011, 2012, 2017

[4] American Council on Exercise Personal Trainer Manual – Fifth Edition

ISBN 978-1-890720-50-6

[5] Added sugars drive Coronary Heart Disease via Insulin Resistance and Hyperinsulinemia: A New Paradigm

Published: 2017

https://openheart.bmj.com/content/4/2/e000729

[6] Insulin Resistance and Alzheimer's Disease: Bioenergetic Linkages

Published: October 2017

https://www.ncbi.nlm.nih.gov/pmc/articles/PMC5671587/

[7] Consuming fructose-sweetened, not glucose sweetened beverages increases visceral adiposity and lipids [*Fat Gain*] and decreased insulin sensitivity [*Increased Insulin Resistance*] in overweight/obese humans

Published: April 2009

https://www.jci.org/articles/view/37385

[8] Effects of Glucose or Fructose Feeding on Glycogen Repletion in Muscle and Liver After Exercise or Fasting

Published: 1987

https://www.ncbi.nlm.nih.gov/pubmed/3592616

[9] Perspective: Protein Requirements and Optimal Intakes in Aging: Are We Ready to Recommend More Than the Recommended Daily Allowance?

Published: May 2018

https://academic.oup.com/advances/article-abstract/9/3/171/4964951

BONUS #1

Don't "Drink" Your Calories

As we have already outlined, the sugar contained in soda, sweet tea, sports drinks, and juices easily adds useless calories.

It also wreaks havoc on your endocrine system by causing massive insulin spikes that end in a crash.

This makes you hungrier and zaps your energy levels. It creates an atmosphere where fat loss is nearly impossible!

Don't be fooled by fruit 'juicing' either. No one needs 2 bananas, 2 pears, and an apple blended into a sugar laden drink!

Blending breaks down the food, causing it to digest faster. This increases the insulin response due to the rapid absorption (bad, if fat loss is the goal or if you're diabetic).

If you want fruit, eat it whole with the fiber intact.

> Note: It's ok to drink low carb/sugar whey protein. Low carb protein drinks can be an effective tool for people who initially find it hard to eat large amounts of meat.

Eat Protein EVERY Meal and Snack

As we touched on earlier, protein is vital for optimal health as amino acids are the building blocks of the human body.

It's important to get enough to ensure muscle preservation as we age and during times of injury or major stressors. It's also needed to support lean muscle growth, which you want.

Additionally, protein dramatically increases your feeling of fullness. This makes overeating difficult.
Fill up on as much as you need to feel satisfied. It should be the main focus of every meal and snack you consume.

As a general target, aim for 20-40 grams of protein at every snack and meal.

A woman at 120 lbs would do well to shoot for 20 grams per meal/snack to total 100+ grams per day.

A man at 200+ lbs would do well to get 35-40 grams per meal/snack to total 170+ grams per day.

These numbers ensure an affective amount for increasing lean mass and keeping hunger at bay.

1oz of meat = about 7 grams of protein...Use this to estimate the protein content of your meal. (i.e. 5 oz of cooked meat = about 35 grams of protein)

Switch to Diet Drinks (If you MUST have them)

Many people are addicted to their favorite beverage. We see this often. They can't imagine giving up their 6 colas per day! This is where we feel it is fine to 'trick' your body and mind...

Replace your sugary drink with a sugar free version.

It will taste different at first, but it is a helpful way to transition yourself away from the harmful sugar.

Many often worry about 'artificial sweetener', but as we have shown; extra sugar causes extreme damage to your body (liver, cardiovascular system, hormones).

A few diet sodas on any given day, are NOT going to have this effect on the body.

I personally used this 'trick' at a young age.

That said, diet soda is still not 'good' for you; so still try to limit to one 12 oz can (maybe 2) per day.

Try to focus on increasing water intake.

Fix One Thing at a Time (NEVER feel hopeless)

We see many people start a new plan, only to quit soon after.

We've seen people drop 20+ lbs, only to revert back to their old habits and gain it all back.

Why would you work so hard, only to let it all slip away from you?

A common theme is the "All or Nothing" mindset. Everyone wants the end result in the shortest amount of time.

That's NOT how any of this works.

You have been lied to by a revolving door of "Magic Pill" and "Fad Diet" marketing.

Here, we only care for truth!

Good health, fat loss, and muscle gain take **long term** effort and consistency. Most make it harder than it needs to be by trying to fix everything at one time.

You can't graduate college with a degree after only one week on campus. It takes time to learn and apply new information.

Take it one day at a time. Progress slowly by changing 1-2 habits at a time. You can only 'fail' if you quit entirely (but you now understand this is NOT an option).

Measure Your Carb Sources

As we have outlined, obesity and related metabolic issues are the result of prolonged 'over-consumption' of carbohydrates. Primarily due to high levels of sugar and fructose in the diet.

Eliminating fructose and sugar, with no other changes will help EVERYONE with fat loss goals.

However, it can still be easy to over eat starchy carb sources like rice and potatoes.

We recommend you measure out your carb sources early on.

Most people do not do well by 'eye-balling' how much rice they have on their plate. 1/2 cup cooked has about 25 carbs (that Chinese takeout you ate likely had at least 1 cup or more).

Do not worry about measuring your meat or veggies. Protein is not easily converted to fat in the body and is of little concern for overconsumption.

If meat were harmful, our ancestors would have been suffering extreme rates of obesity and diabetes (they didn't).

They ate tons of meat but did not suffer the metabolic issues we do today!

If you're hungry, fill up on these items. The meat keeps you fuller longer and protein is essential for good health and sense of well-being!

Plan Your Meals (Prep in advance)

Don't get stuck in a situation where you have to settle for food that doesn't fit your goals.

Prepare large batches of your favorite meat and veggies at one time, for the week.

Boil a big pot of sweet potatoes and refrigerate for a quick side later.

Hard boil eggs for the week as a snack/breakfast item.

Buy a Crockpot. Get creative!

Have fun and pick the healthy food you love. Don't force yourself to eat broccoli if you hate it!

A "Calorie is NOT a Calorie"

For many decades, mainstream health and government agencies have preached that a "calorie is a calorie". This is one of the tragic myths that keep people from reaching their goals.

Imagine the following:

Person #1: Eats 2000 calories of only ribeye, every day for a month.

Person #2: Eats 2000 calories of only cookies, every day for a month.

I can assure you, these 2 individuals will have dramatically different results.

Person #1 will lose body fat and likely have high energy levels, due to maintaining a low and controlled blood sugar.

Person #2 will experience a roller coaster of blood sugar spikes and crashes. They are constantly filling up the buckets (as described earlier) of their liver and muscle cells; constantly driving excess sugar into their fat cells.

This person is hungry and is never satisfied from a meal. A vicious cycle, and no way to live!

So NO, a calorie, is NOT a calorie!

The types of calories we consume, drastically changes how we process and use them.

This means that a calorie in, is not a "calorie out"...

The 2000 calories of ribeye will be used to support energy needs, but the body will also use it for 'new protein production' and 'new bone production', due to its high protein and natural fat content.

This means, more of these calories are used for optimizing the body...rather than being stored as fat. The body has many ways it can use the extra calories rather than simply storing them in the fat cells!

Said another way...

Calories "out" are DEPENDENT on calories in!

(2000 calories from cookies is useless to the body, and it quickly stores it as fat!)

By following a natural whole food diet high in meat (protein) and veggies, moderate in healthy fats, with some natural carb sources (just enough to support training), you will never struggle with weight again.

STOP counting calories and choose natural foods.

These healthy calories are far more likely to be used by the body, rather than stored as fat.

When you do this, the body will regulate itself overtime, and will tell you when you are 'actually' hungry (high sugar intake throws off these normal processes).

I personally count my protein intake (to ensure I get the minimum amount I need) and keep track of how many carbs I have consumed (when in doubt I keep them low).

Before you eat it, ask, "How will this food affect my body?"

We are brainwashed and tricked into choosing foods based on emotion and convenience!

You now choose food based on how it will affect you!

Is what you are about to eat going to help you reach your goals, or hurt them?

Will it help you live longer? Will it help your joint pain and inflammation?

Will this food make your health issues worse?

Are you in control of your choices? **OR** …

Are you letting food control your choices?

You have all the information you need to make an informed decision now!

You don't need to be perfect!

You just need to start thinking about how food is going to help or hurt you in your pursuit of a stronger and healthier life!

If you have a bad meal or a bad eating day…follow it up with a good day!

Over time…You will have more good days than bad days.

This is when lasting change can occur!

'Over Eat' Protein to Lose Weight (Don't Count Calories)

Counting calories is **NOT** a long-term strategy.

When you drop calories to a low level like many 1000-1200 calorie diets call for, **your metabolism resets** itself by slowing down to keep you from losing any more weight.

NOTE: The metabolism drops with **prolonged** low-calorie diets (over weeks, not days). So if you ever try 24 hour 'fasting', this will not shut down your metabolism. Fasting is used as a short term healthy break from food. After any fast, however, you should return to a normal eating pattern and caloric intake!

This is why many people do well for 4-6 weeks but get frustrated when the weight and fat loss stalls.

Most times, people do not take in enough protein, so when they lose weight from a calorie restricted diet, they are losing fat AND muscle.

Here's the kicker…

Then they go back to eating like they were previously (higher calorie and higher carb), but NOW their metabolism is slower.

Therefore, they easily gain back ALL the weight lost, but what is gained back is nearly all fat and not the muscle that's been lost!

They are no better off than they were!

Here is the SOLUTION:

Eat as much protein (& veggies) as you can. Eat until you can't eat any more.

When you do this, over time, you will find it easier to avoid the craving for junk food, because you will be full and satisfied from your previous meal.

This will help you **snack less**! You will find it hard to "overeat" because meat takes longer to digest!

I have used this strategy for over 15 years. It is one way I keep myself from overeating processed junk food. I have found it extremely useful in managing my weight for the last decade and a half.

So... Eat all the meat, eggs, fish, and 'low starch' veggies you desire! Pick your favorites!

Get creative with spices and different flavors (avoid sugary sauces though).

Then it will be harder to over eat processed junk food!

You DO NOT Need 6 Meals per Day

Here's a secret...

Eating 6 meals per day, does NOT 'increase' your metabolism!

It does however, tend to make you hungrier and often you will tend to eat more calories throughout the day, without noticing! (I'm speaking from experience.)

If you are not hungry, you do not have to eat!

When you get on a whole food (low processed food) lifestyle, you will find that hunger **regulates itself!**

You will often be able to go 6-8 hours between meals, and guess what, this does not shut down your metabolism.

BUT you still do need to make sure you aren't eating 'too little' (Keep the metabolism going).

Again, it's important to eat plenty of protein (6+ ounces), veggies, and some healthier fats as the main focus of your meals.

(And some low glycemic natural carbs sources in smaller amounts depending on your specific goal).

BONUS #2

Create a VISION of Where You Want to Be (and never be a victim)

This is important. You must imagine the body and life you desire. Do you want 6-pack abs, or to simply feel stronger and more energetic?

You must stop any negative thoughts about why you can't reach your vision...

If you don't, you are setting yourself up to fail before you begin.

Set your vision, build a positive mindset towards it (You cannot fail).

This creates the atmosphere needed for you to stay in the game long enough to reach your vision.

The problem for most is NOT genetics or time. The issue is they don't believe enough in themselves to see their vision through.

We believe in you, why shouldn't you?

Take Control, Take Action...Reach your Vision!

Choose Whether You Live a Dream or a Nightmare

Your mind can NOT tell the difference between what you imagine and what is real!

"Visualization" in the mind is a very REAL and POWERFUL skill to practice.

Think of a dream or a nightmare...

You are asleep and ALL of what's happening is in your mind!

If you had a good dream, you likely wake up feeling relaxed and energized!

If you had a bad dream, you likely wake up in a cold sweat with your heart pounding!

What is DIFFERENT?
You were asleep...You didn't do anything "physical"!
So the end result (nervous sweat vs. energized well-being) ...
Is ALL in the MIND!

YOUR own mind literally controlled how you felt physically...

Most people don't think this way, mainly because they have never been taught to.

I assure you, the people who learn to leverage the power of their own minds are the ones who will have the greatest success in any field or goal...

1.) Visualize winning in your mind, **first**!
2.) Build a mental movie of **how** you are going to win!
3.) Feel what victory will be like. **Smell** it...**Taste** it...**See** it...**Hear** it!

Practice Winning in your mind, for YOUR:

- **Health/Fitness Goals** (What steps are required for Fat Loss and Better Health?)
- **Social Interactions** (What should I work on to make meeting new people, easier?)
- **Business** (How can I create more value?)
- **Family** (How I can I help them prosper?)
- **Job** (How can I add value, and be worth a higher income?)
- **Money** (What is the best use of my funds? How can I get ahead financially?)

What are the answers to these questions?

That depends on the person. It depends on YOU!

Everyone has a different background. NO ONE has experienced the exact same life as you.

Your situation could be similar to others (but never the same) ...

Dig deep into your mind and find the answers...

Re-read the questions in the list above...

They are a starting point to help you begin thinking in a different way!

Always start with

> **"How can I...."**
> **"What can I..."**

Anytime you start a thought or phrase with "I can't...", you are 100% correct! You have already shut your mind off to the possibility of winning! **(You must avoid this.)**

Be affirmative and positive, start visualizing HOW winning feels; and WHAT you must do to win!

YOU get to decide whether you live a "dream" or if you live a "nightmare"...

It starts in your mind!

Re-Program Your Mind

I repeat again, your mind is a powerful thing. If you do not work to **re-program** 'how you think', I promise you will never have lasting results.

Many people do very well for weeks and months, but usually, their underlying 'Mindsets' have never been trained or addressed.

This makes you susceptible to relapse.

Just like a drug addict, who turns back to the needle after gaining sobriety. Your mind is a computer program! Your habits are the "Code" that runs it.

Therefore, you must re-program your daily habits and thinking, to improve how your computer performs!

Do you want LASTING CHANGE?

Then you must work as hard on your 'Mind', as you do your 'Body'.

You will fail if you don't fix your thinking...

> (I must be blunt here, because I've seen too many people walk away when they are on the edge of a major breakthrough. I will not allow YOU, to fall into this trap. You are in control, so never except defeat. Your future self depends on your present self!)

So, how do you do this?

I will give a start...BUT, you must practice building your own "Mindset Shifts"...

Study these closely...

CHANGE:

"I choose food by how it tastes"→ **"I choose by how it affects me"**
"My genetics hold me back" → **"I am holding myself back"**
"I can't find a way" → **"I will make a way"**
"I don't have time" → **"I must make time"**
"Being healthy is hard" → **"I refuse to die of a disease"**
"My kids need me home" → **"My kids need me to live longer"**
"You only live once" → **"I must maximize my only life"**

What you "THINK", is a "CHOICE"!

How will you make better choices?

Now, allow me to continue with some helpful honesty…

Everything is Your Responsibility to Attack (Take back control of YOUR life)

It's your responsibility to fix it. No one is coming to save the day.

There is no 'knight in shining armor'.

Life doesn't work that way. Unfortunately, society has lied to us. We are on our own.

The honest truth is…

If you don't like it, YOU must change it.

There are people who can help along the way (Like Jessica and I), but your life is YOURS to lead!

So what if…

> Someone said 'mean' things to you?
> **IGNORE THEM** (If you don't, they control you)
>
> You tried, but failed?
> **TRY AGAIN!** (With a better plan)
>
> You don't know how?
> **FIGURE IT OUT!** (Winners find a way…YOU ARE ONE!)

I could go on, but you get the point. YOU are the one who controls your mind and body.

YOU decide what you think about and focus on. YOU, YOU, YOU…

If you think negative thoughts, you will become a negative person. Think positive thoughts, you become a positive person.

What you THINK about, you WILL become!
(Very important to remember this)

Drown yourself in positivity for a while. (Hard to do in today's world.)

If this means you only listen to 'self-help' books in the car instead of music, then so be it. (I highly recommend this by the way.)

It's time to immerse yourself with positive thoughts, positive books or podcasts, and positive people.

Avoid all the negativity you can for a while and see what a difference it makes in your life.

I am not saying to walk around with a dopey weird smile all day…

But making an effort to remove negativity from your life will drastically improve your mood and well-being!

We are only interested in seeing you SUCCEED with your individual goals.

We refuse to let you fall into the negative traps many people make.

We can't do it FOR you…but we know YOU are capable of taking control and living a stronger life!

May God bless you and lead you on your journey!

BONUS #3

(To be used as secondary tools)

We left any discussion about supplementation to the end of this guide!

Why?

Because your lifestyle (food choices and exercise) are the **MOST** important thing to correct!

We are tired of people wasting money and time on short-term diet pills, ineffective programs, and falling victim to clever marketing tricks.

Supplements are only a "TOOL" that can be used to enhance your results.

In this section, we cover the basics we believe everyone should consider as part of their pursuit in optimizing their bodies and health!

> [Disclaimer: We are not doctors and we are not "prescribing" any of these items to you! You should obviously discuss any supplements you take with your doctor to be sure there are no adverse reactions to medications you may already be on.
>
> Everything we list here is 'natural' in origin, and we personally take each of these items on a daily basis. You must decide for yourself what is right for you!]

Multi-Vitamin

Many believe that you can get by with no extra vitamins if you eat healthy. In my experience, I have a greater feeling of well-being when I regularly take a multi-vitamin. My energy levels and immune system seem to be noticeably elevated.

Being deficient in certain vitamins and minerals can have a negative effect on your fat loss and weight management goals. Many of these elements are vital to proper production and balance of your hormone levels.

A quality vitamin supplement is a good insurance policy, to ensure your body has everything it needs to optimize itself! (Assuming you've corrected your diet as a 1st line treatment.)

Vitamin D3

The truth is, Vitamin D isn't actually a vitamin...It's a hormone the body uses for many important functions! With our busy, indoor lifestyles (lack of sunlight), many people are deficient in this important hormone.

This can have a significant impact on your mood, anxiety levels, and over all sense of well-being.

The common recommendation to ensure adequate intake is between...

5000-10000 IU dosage of vitamin D3 daily.

Fish Oil

Omega 3 fatty acids are another important contributor to the bodies hormonal balance.

It's difficult to get enough Omega 3 in our diets. Certain types of fish are the ultimate source, but one must be aware of mercury levels in certain species.

1-3 grams daily of EPA/DHA in fish oil capsules is an easy way to increase your intake.

(Only count the milligrams dose from EPA/DHA on the label. EPA/DHA is where the majority of the health benefits lie. Many brands will market a product as "1200 mg Fish Oil", but look closer and it only has 300 mg of EPA/DHA)

Omega 3 intake is linked to lower rates of cardiovascular disease. The Japanese as an example, have some of the highest intake per capita, and experience some of the lowest rates of heart disease!

Omega 3 is also helpful in your quest to reduce inflammation. Long term use, can be helpful with minor joint pain. I notice a slight decrease in knee pain when I take regular doses of 2-3 grams daily.

Magnesium

Magnesium is an essential mineral that many tend to be deficient in. If you suffer routinely from cramping in your hands, feet, or other areas of the body it's possible you have a mineral imbalance or possibly a low level of magnesium.

Consider adding a few magnesium capsules per day, or even just an occasional Epsom Salt bath (a relaxing option).

Low levels of magnesium can also contribute to higher levels of anxiety, insomnia, and fatigue; so, it makes sense to ensure you maintain a minimum level needed by the body.

Whey Protein

Whey is a supplement that has been used in the bodybuilding and fitness industry for many years.

I have personally used whey as part of my regular diet for the last 15 years. I find that I get less run down and recover better from weight training when I add 1-2 scoops per day after training and/or between meals.

When I am consistent with it as a "TOOL" in my diet, I also find that I rarely get sick (presumably from the immune boosting effects of the amino acids).

I also use it routinely as a way to get more protein into my diet, without adding a ton of extra calories.

Many people have found it useful as a way to overcome cravings between meals. The higher levels of amino acids (protein) in whey helps to trigger a feeling of satiety (reduced hunger).

If you are weight training regularly, I find it even more helpful as a tool to get high quality protein in after intense training.

Many people find it hard to eat immediately after a hard workout, so 1-2 scoops after training is helpful to jumpstart recovery.

I've tried not taking whey for periods of time, but always go back to it, because I can tell a difference in my recovery and how I feel.

What to look for:

The highest quality whey proteins are "cold-processed" "hydrolyzed" "Isolates". The higher quality products tend to cost a bit more, but they also mix easier and taste much better in my experience.

In general, 1 scoop of whey should contain approximately 20-25 grams of protein and total about 100 to 150 calories.

Your cheaper quality brands will be predominately whey protein "concentrate" or blends of concentrate and isolate. These are still quality sources of protein, but in my experience the taste and mixing ability are lacking.

If you are sensitive to 'lactose' a quality whey isolate will be a better option for you, as nearly all of the lactose is removed.

It really comes down to quality, purity, taste, & ease of mixing.

Many of the major supplement brands on store shelves are cheaper, lower quality versions.

They are decent options for protein content, but you should find a product you like the taste and quality of. This way, it is a better "tool" for you to use as an 'in between' meal option.

If you hate the taste, you won't use it! (This is the most common complaint I've heard.)

Berberine (Natural Alternative to Diabetes Prescription Metformin)

Have you heard of this herb? Probably not!

Its origins come from its use in ancient Chinese medicine but has been overlooked in modern health practice!

Berberine is just now gaining more attention for its blood sugar lowering ability.

You may be familiar with Metformin, which is a diabetic pharmaceutical that has been used for decades in the treatment of diabetes and elevated blood sugar levels.

Combined with a lower sugar/carbohydrate diet, Metformin is effective in reversing Insulin Resistance (discussed earlier).

One study compared the effects of Metformin to that of Berberine in separate groups of diabetic patients. They found that Berberine was just as effective as Metformin in lowering blood sugar levels.

In addition, they noted that Berberine had a beneficial effect on triglyceride and cholesterol levels that Metformin did not; and it significantly helped improve 'insulin sensitivity' (meaning it lowered insulin resistance...**VERY GOOD for fat loss**).

REFERENCE:
Efficacy of Berberine in Patients with Type 2 Diabetes https://www.ncbi.nlm.nih.gov/pmc/articles/PMC2410097/#!po=22.3684

Berberine is also shown to help promote better body fat loss in the mid-section. I'm not saying it is a "magic pill" but it is a "tool' to consider in addition to your lifestyle change and better food choices.

In combination with a quality diet, Berberine, appears to be a strong alternative for those who wish to better control blood sugar and enhance fat loss results!

Since I have added it to my own supplement routine, I have noticed some benefit in reducing stubborn belly fat!

Dosage: 1500 mg daily... spread across the day. (i.e. One 500mg pill at breakfast/lunch/dinner)

Supplement Summary:

Again, supplements are only a "tool" to help you reach your weight and fat-loss goals.

The listed supplements are some of the priorities any one should be able to safely take (just remember to discuss with your doctor, to be sure).

We personally use each of these supplements to help OPTIMIZE our bodies and our hormone levels.

Stop wasting money on special "magic pills" and cover your bases with quality vitamins and targeted supplements like Whey and Berberine!

Eat a high quality natural diet as much as possible. Work every day to be better, and never get discouraged. THEN, use supplements as a "tool".

We often get asked what specific supplements we (Jessica & Bradley) use...

This section lays out the specific health supplements we use for optimum health!

For Vitamin D3 and Magnesium, you should be good with several different brands. These are cheap and generally effective in my experience.

For Fish Oil and Berberine, it is important to find a reputable trusted brand/manufacturer. (This really applies to all supplements, so do some research to pay attention to the EPA/DHA for Fish Oil.)

We personally use "Micro Factor" (It's an All in One Full Spectrum Vitamin/Mineral Supplement) and whey protein from 1stPhorm. We do actually use their fish oil as well.

I don't usually recommend specific brands; however, I have found the quality and taste of their whey protein products to be far superior to the countless popular mainstream brands I've tried. (I truly stand by this statement.)

Because of this, it is the only brand we display at "Goins Strong Fitness".

We would never recommend any product that we did not personally use ourselves and could speak to its quality or efficacy.

If you would like to check out the vitamins and/or protein, receive Free Shipping, and a 110% Money Back Guarantee...make sure to use the link below:

www.1stPhorm.com/GoinsStrong

Fasting Guide:

How Skipping Meals Can Benefit you!
BONUS #4

I already know what you're thinking..."These people are telling me to starve myself to lose weight"...

Let me be clear. Intermittent Fasting or Fasting in general is NOT a starvation plan.

It is simply the idea of giving yourself a break from food to allow the body to properly regulate itself, without the constant bombardment of digesting food.

This time away from food can help lower insulin levels in the body, when used properly. No food and/or insulin spiking carbohydrates are ingested, so insulin levels have a chance to dramatically decrease.

(Good news if you are currently overweight and insulin resistant.)

Mainstream advice of eating 6 smalls meals a day, is a late 20th century idea!

Is this advice working?... **70% of Americans are overweight or obese!**

Seems to me, this mainstream advice is hurting Americans…not helping!

Our ancestors did not eat 6 times per day, because they understood it was not necessary and they didn't have 24/7 access to food.

They relied on hunting game as a primary food source, as meat and protein are vital for proper functioning of the body.

In times of abundant meat, they would eat large amounts because it might be a day or more before the next successful hunt!

Our bodies are designed to go for long periods of time without food. It actually has several benefits that come with it.

The mainstream belief is that skipping breakfast or any other meal, will slow your metabolism (NOT TRUE).

The other major belief is that skipping meals makes you eat more later in the day. This is somewhat true.

If you are used to eating a highly processed American diet and you already struggle to make good food choices, then you will tend to over-indulge in those same items late in the day. (Like eating a whole bag of chips) ...

The key is to eat whole natural foods, like we laid out earlier in Part 2.

Eating these natural foods makes it more difficult to over-eat later in the day, because the size and bulk of the whole food meal is more hunger satisfying than a family size bag of chips.

The issue is not skipping meals, the issue is making poor food choices when you are starving. Be aware of this and avoid reaching for that bag of processed junk.

Now, allow me to shift direction a bit...

For several years I have played around with "carb-timing", which I view as a form of Intermittent Fasting.

Basically, I typically eat carbs once or twice per day.

At lunch on weight training days, and in my post workout meal.

I never eat carbs in the morning (just protein and some fat). I have done this for many years and find it easier to stay lean than when I followed a standard diet consuming carbs at each meal.

I also noticed I had more consistent energy levels and better focus. This is presumably from the steady blood sugar levels it helps to maintain.

I call this "Intermittent Carb Fasting"...I don't know if anyone else has coined this phrase. If not, I claim it here.

But this is not "true" fasting, as I typically eat plenty of protein and healthy fat in the morning hours.

True fasting is going without food entirely. This also means any drinkable calories, which you learned to avoid in the "Tips & Advice" section earlier.

Here are the most common fasting strategies:

16/8 Fasting: Here, you fast for 16 hours every day and restrict eating to an eight (8) hour window (ex. 12PM to 8PM).

Basically, this is just skipping breakfast and not eating before bed. This is the version that I practice myself on the regular basis.

I always make sure to keep my calorie intake at normal levels, so my lunch and dinner meals are larger than on a 6 meal per day plan. Servings of meat are typically around 8oz + at lunch and dinner.

One meal per day: With this strategy, you pick one or two days of the week and fast for 24 hours, from dinner one night until dinner the next day; eating nothing in between.

There are people who do this every day, but this is extreme for anyone just starting to consider the idea of fasting.

This is not 'low calorie' though. The idea is to eat your normal calorie intake. If you eat 2000 calories on normal days, then you would try to eat close to that.

If you do it only occasionally, then falling too low in calories won't drop your metabolism.

5:2 Diet: This is a more advanced strategy for fasting. Five days of the week, you eat normally.

Then, for the remaining two days you fast. Consuming no more than 500–600 calories those days, even more advanced...No calories at all!

There are many thousands of people... Millions if we consider religious based fasting... who regularly restrict or time their food without shutting down their metabolisms.

The more I practice fasting, the faster I have been able to drop belly fat. My results are consistent with the research and the accounts of many other individuals.

I'm not sure why these strategies have not become more mainstream, but I assure you it will in the years to come. The benefits are astounding when you dig into the existing research.

Here are some of the MAJOR benefits of Intermittent Fasting:

1) Blood Sugar Control and Reduced Insulin Resistance

I lead with this, because it is the basis of this guide. Controlling blood sugar and insulin is the key to long term fat loss and overall good health.

Intermittent Fasting is a major weapon to help you accomplish this goal.

While fasting, your body gets a chance to properly regulate itself. Insulin levels are reduced in the body and blood sugar levels are kept at a lower level.

Anything that helps accomplish a lower blood sugar and reduces insulin levels, is beneficial in preventing insulin resistance and diabetes; and will also benefit the heart and cardiovascular system (as we outlined in Part 1 of this guide).

Human studies have found intermittent fasting helps reduce fasting blood sugar, and fasting insulin. [1]

How large this affect is will vary from person to person, but it is now well established that intermittent fasting has positive benefits in blood sugar regulation.

2) Fasting Positively Affects Cell Function and Hormones

Several great hormonal and bodily processes occur when we go without eating:

- Insulin levels drop, enhancing weight loss results. [2]
- Growth Hormone increases [3]
- Cell repair process increases (removing cellular waste) [4]

These are just a few of the benefits, and each of these are beneficial to anyone struggling with fat-loss and insulin resistance!

Giving your body a break from processed or inflammatory food, appears to have a profound affect in helping it achieve a normal hormonal balance.

The body seems to get a chance to focus on healing itself, rather than recovering from poor quality food intake.

3) Fasting is Good for the Brain

As we have established, controlling blood sugar and lowering insulin resistance will help reduce inflammation in the body.

This means that your vascular system (blood vessels and arteries) are less inflamed as well. The side effect of this is better 'blood flow'!

The brain is often overlooked as part of this overall system, BUT…

The brain is directly affected by blood flow and inflammation in the body. This affects your ability to focus, how you think, and ultimately how you feel.

Anything that reduces inflammation, and increases blood flow, will greatly benefit the brain.

There are established studies in rats that show intermittent fasting may increase the growth of new nerve cells, and this would have direct benefits for brain function. [5]

From personal experience, I can tell you that Intermittent Fasting in the morning helps me focus and stay more productive.

Once you adjust to not eating in the morning hunger pains won't typically pick up until around lunch time.

4) Fasting May Help Extend Lifespan

This is one of the more promising possibilities for Intermittent Fasting. It is known that calorie restriction may have positive affects in increasing lifespan in humans. [6]

Intermittent Fasting (eating in a short window <8 hours) induces some of the same effects as 'calorie restriction' even though calories are not necessarily reduced day to day.

This could make Intermittent Fasting a tool for life extension.

It will be many years before any definite study comes out confirming any claims on life extension, however, the positive affects induced by Intermittent Fasting are significant and plentiful.

When all the data is viewed collectively, it makes sense to conclude that fasting will not hurt your desire to live a longer life.

CONCLUSION:

Remember, Fasting is NOT a starvation or 'calorie restriction' plan!

However, eating in a time restricted window makes it difficult to overeat.

It can be helpful for anyone who struggles with constant hunger…

If you can overcome the urge to eat many times per day, the body begins to regulate hunger at a normal level.

Constantly eating high carb, processed food, makes you THINK you are constantly hungry because of how it negatively affects the body.

Giving your body a break from excessive food on the regular basis will help you overcome a constant urge to eat.

Of course, this also happens when you switch to a more natural whole food diet, as we have outlined.

Play around with intermittent fasting every now and then. Skip carbs in the morning and just eat protein and healthy fat (several eggs for example).

Then take a step further and skip breakfast entirely one day. Then eat a healthy lunch as you normally would.

Start with one (1) day a week, if you give it a try. Then try two (2) days. Continue and see what differences you notice for yourself.

Men and Women can be different here, and how you feel initially can vary greatly between individuals.

If you are diabetic and take insulin, make sure you keep a close eye on your blood sugar levels, as you could accidentally allow blood sugar to drop too low. As always, consult with your doctor.

Blood sugar levels in healthy individuals will properly regulate and will not drop too low.

Good luck in your pursuit of a longer and stronger life!

References

[1] Intermittent fasting vs daily calorie restriction for type 2 diabetes prevention: a review of human findings
https://www.sciencedirect.com/science/article/pii/S193152441400200X

[2] Alternate-day fasting in nonobese subjects: effects on body weight, body composition, and energy metabolism.
https://www.ncbi.nlm.nih.gov/pubmed/15640462

[3] Augmented growth hormone (GH) secretory burst frequency and amplitude mediate enhanced GH secretion during a two-day fast in normal men.
https://www.ncbi.nlm.nih.gov/pubmed/1548337

[4] Short-term fasting induces profound neuronal autophagy
https://www.ncbi.nlm.nih.gov/pmc/articles/PMC3106288/

[5] Dietary restriction increases the number of newly generated neural cells, and induces BDNF expression, in the dentate gyrus of rats.
https://www.ncbi.nlm.nih.gov/pubmed/11220789

[6] Calorie restriction and aging: review of the literature and implications for studies in humans
https://academic.oup.com/ajcn/article/78/3/361/4689958

Made in United States
Cleveland, OH
05 November 2026

47653968R00040